Intermittent Fasting

A Guide To Getting Started

sources. Please consult a licensed professional before attempting any techniques outlined in this book.

By reading this document, the reader agrees that under no circumstances is the author responsible for any losses, direct or indirect, which are incurred as a result of the use of information contained within this document, including, but not limited to, —errors, omissions, or inaccuracies.

Table of Contents

Introduction

I want to thank you and congratulate you for purchasing this book, *"Intermittent Fasting: A Guide To Getting Started"* I hope you find it informative in your quest to learn about intermittent fasting and how it will help you transform your life.

On the road to good health, we often face few obstacles every now and then; that delicious cake filled with cream cheese frosting or those mouthwatering nachos with cheese and beans that you were craving for. It can get hard for us to lose weight and remain strong and healthy. What do we do then? We hit the gym, work extra hard and get that body into shape just in time for the big wedding or reunion so we don't feel bad about the weight. But then what happens after the wedding? The cycle stays the same.

We get back to our daily routine and forget about everything that we need to do to remain fit and healthy. Demotivated by the weight gain, we believe it was the fault of that one slice of pizza or cake that we ate the night before. This will make you hate the way you look, which can lead to some serious health issues – mental and physical.

I bet you have tried different diets to compensate for the lack of exercise. There are numerous diets like the Ketogenic diet, General Motors diet, Paleo diet and many more. Since each of these diets was designed for a certain type of body, it becomes difficult to choose the diet that works best for your body. These diets also ask you to avoid some food groups since those groups will lead to weight gain. So, how can you decide which of these diets will work for you? If you do not want to follow any diet, but want to make changes to your lifestyle, then this book is designed just for you. This book will open doors into a new world of health and happiness.

Intermittent fasting is not an extreme form of diet and was followed by our ancestors. The idea of intermittent fasting involves a cycle of eating periods and fasting periods, which force the body to rely on the fat that is stored in the body. The body will burn this fat to provide different organs with energy. In this book, you can find different types of Intermittent Fasting, which are followed by millions across the world. With record stated benefits for this type of a diet, it is one of the most widely accepted forms of diet that does not restrict you from consuming your favorite dishes.

In this book, you will learn how you can design the perfect diet for your body without giving up on your favorite food. Over the course of this book, you will learn about the different types of Intermittent Fasting. You can then choose one that fits your needs and start your journey toward a healthy and happy life.

This book is a guide into the world of leading a healthier lifestyle with a sneak peek into the benefits of following an Intermittent Fasting diet. It also answers the most pressing questions that people have regarding this diet.

Are you excited to start your fitness journey? If yes then, without any further ado, let us get started and learn more about intermittent fasting.

Thanks again for purchasing this book, I hope you enjoy it!

Chapter One: An Introduction to Intermittent Fasting

When you hear the term fasting, there will be by default a negative outlook towards it. Staying away from food is not at all an interesting prospect. But did you know that you fast every day for at least 8 hours? Did that take you by surprise? If you do not think this is true – think about it. You consume your first meal after having slept for eight hours. You consume breakfast because you want to do exactly what the name says – "break the fast." That is almost how Intermittent Fasting works. The concept of intermittent fasting is not new but has been around for thousands of years. In this chapter, you will gather information on the science behind intermittent fasting.

Before diving into the actuals of intermittent fasting, you must know the difference between the terms "fed state" and "fasting state." On any given day, when we consume food, our body will convert solid foods into glucose. It will then break glucose down into glycogen. This compound is stored in the liver or in the muscles. How does this happen? Well, the body produces an important component that aids in the conversion process called "insulin." Insulin is a hormone that regulates the levels of glucose in the body. Insulin is a protein that helps the body store the glycogen in the liver.

Since insulin can only store a limited amount of carbohydrates in the liver, the surplus is then converted into fat and stored in the muscle. This is what contributes to weight gain. Our body automatically stores glucose in the liver. If there is a surplus of glucose in our body, the glucose that is accessible and can be used immediately is stored in the liver and that which is harder to access is stored in the muscle.

In Intermitted fasting, you do not force your body to starve. When your body switches into the starvation mode, it will become difficult to calculate your caloric intake. In an intermittent fasting eating pattern, you provide your body with the necessary nutrition, but also allow your body to shift into the fasting state. Normally followed in the ratio of 16:8 where an individual eats for 8 hours in the day and fast for 16 hours, Intermittent Fasting helps the body to forcibly access the extra fat stored in the muscle and use it for its energy/fuel.

This method will help you train your mind to crave less. You can also train your mind to reduce your hunger pangs. This will give your body a chance to live off of the stored fat in the body. While there are several who go by this kind of eating lifestyle and swear by its benefits, there are no proven reports about the side effects of the diet, if any.

Chapter Two: Benefits of Intermittent Fasting

There are many benefits to following the intermittent fasting eating pattern. Let us look at some of these benefits.

Changes in Metabolism

The intermittent fasting eating pattern will change your metabolism in the following ways:

Drop in Insulin:

During the fed state, the body will release insulin, which will work on storing the glucose. While fasting, the insulin levels drop which sends the body a signal to use the stored fat to provide fuel to the organs. This helps to facilitate weight loss.

Increase in Human Growth Hormone:

During the fasting state, the body releases the growth hormone (HGH). This hormone plays a key role in burning the fat in the body. It will also aid in muscle growth.

Noradrenaline:

During the fasting state the nervous system sends signals to the fat cells in the body using a hormone called Noradrenaline. This hormone converts the stored fat into fatty acids that are used by the body as fuel

Changes in Weight

Studies show that intermittent fasting helps you lose up to 3-8% of your body fat in a 3- 24-week period. When you follow this eating pattern, you will automatically reduce your caloric intake. You will also start eating healthy food. This will help your body focus on repairing any damage.

Consume a Balanced Diet

Since the feeding window for the body is not more than 8 hours, the number of meals you can accommodate in this period can be no more than two. These two meals must be packed with all the necessary nutrients. It is difficult to plan and stick to such a diet, but it becomes easy with meal prep. This also means more time in hand, which allows you to work on your many hobbies.

Reduces Type-2 Diabetes

With the advent of fast food centers and ready to eat dishes, people have begun to consume more than what is deemed necessary. In the past, people could consume delicious and healthy food for just $1. Companies like Mc Donald's, however, have changed the face of eating. Due to the consumption of foods that are high in sugar and salt, people are at a higher risk of developing Type 2 Diabetes. In the US, close to 30.4 million people have been diagnosed with Type 2 diabetes. With the insulin prices on the rise, the need for following a healthy diet has become even more important. Since following an intermittent fasting lifestyle lowers your insulin levels and blood sugar levels, it is possible to control the effects of Type 2 diabetes.

Automatic Calorie Restriction

When your body is accustomed to fasting, you will automatically reduce your caloric intake. This is due to the fact that you will learn to train your mind into controlling your cravings. You will also begin to consume healthy food that will keep you full for longer. This means that you will need to choose foods that contain high amounts of proteins, good fats and carbohydrates are of priority.

Reduces Inflammation

The human body is designed to fight any kind of illness. The immune system will fight the bad cells in the body, and this activity can lead to inflammation. If different glands in the body begin to inflame, it can open up doors for serious illnesses that can damage the body. Inflammation sometimes causes our cells to attack healthy cells instead of foreign bodies. This leads to some damage. Some of the diseases caused by inflammation are heart problems, stroke and autoimmune diseases such as rheumatoid arthritis and lupus. Intermittent fasting helps reduce this inflammation and makes the body more stable against such illnesses.

Reduces Heart Stroke

Over the last few decades, people have started to consume food that is rich in trans-fat and saturated fat, as this type of food is readily available. The fats in these foods block the arteries, which lead to heart diseases. When you follow the intermittent fasting eating pattern, you will need to choose different food groups that are good for your body. The food that you consume will also help your body heal.

Chapter Three: Who Should Avoid Intermittent Fasting

Experts suggest that some people should not follow the intermittent fasting eating pattern.

Pregnant Women

The calorie requirement is different for pregnant women when compared to other individuals, as pregnant women need to keep themselves and their baby healthy. They are required to consume at least 2,400 calories a day, and it is for this reason that this pattern is not good for them to follow.

Eating Disorders

Individuals with eating disorders can have a very hard time with intermittent fasting. People with an eating disorder either binge or avoid food. This means that they may overeat when they break their fast or not eat at all. This will damage the body.

Children

The human body can function well only when it is provided with the required nutrition. It is essential that children below the age of eighteen are provided with sufficient nutrition since they are naturally active. Experts recommend that this eating pattern should be followed by children who are obese, only if their physicians recommend it.

History of High Stress

Stress is often the root cause of eating disorders. When someone is under a lot of stress, he or she may choose to consume a lot of food. It is hard for people under immense stress to follow the intermittent fasting eating pattern because they will need to restrict themselves from binging on 'comfort food.'

Chapter Four: Types of Intermittent Fasting

The intermittent fasting eating pattern is easy to follow since there are no strict guidelines that you need to follow. You can modify the pattern based on your lifestyle. When you follow this eating pattern, you can save your costs and also ensure that you consume healthy food. This food will ensure that you remain full for longer periods of time. You can always test each pattern and see which one works best for you. All you need to remember is that you should avoid consuming meals or any food during the fasting period. There are some exceptions if you choose to follow the long duration fasting methods instead of the short duration fasting methods. We will cover both types of patterns in this chapter.

The Short Duration Fasting is as follows

12 Hour Fasting

This pattern is also called the regular fasting pattern since we often fast for at least twelve hours anyway. In this pattern, both the eating and fasting windows are for twelve hours. In the eating window, you can consume three whole meals, but avoid snacking in between those meals. The outcome of this pattern is based on the food that you consume during your eating period. You should follow this pattern only if you do not consume any processed food. You can only see the results of this eating pattern if you stick to healthy food.

16/8 Method

Most people follow this pattern. As the name suggests, you will need to fast for sixteen hours and break the fast with an eight-hour eating window. You can adjust your eight-hour eating window depending on your eating habits. For instance, if you are not a breakfast person, you can consume your first meal in the afternoon and end your day with a meal at 8 p.m. If you are a morning person and enjoy your morning breakfast, you can adjust your feeding window accordingly. You should, however, restrict from binging on any junk food. You can consume beverages like water, tea and coffee during your fasting period. You must ensure that you do not consume any aerated or sweetened drinks. This method will not work for you if you break your fast by consuming a large number of calories. Consume food high in good fats and protein-based foods if you want to revive your body and repair any damages.

20:4 Warrior Fasting

This is an extreme short-duration eating pattern. If you want to follow this eating pattern, you should ensure that you have immense will power. You should also learn to listen to your body and give it all the nutrients it needs. As the name suggests, you will need to fast for twenty hours and consume food only in a four-hour eating period. Therefore, you have to choose your meals very wisely. It is always a good idea to prepare the meal yourself since it will give you complete control of what you put into the food. During the 20-hour fasting period, you are not allowed to consume any junk or high-calorie food. You should also avoid binging on junk when you break your fast. Your body will crave for a lot of food during the eating period, and you should ensure that you do not consume food rich in trans-fats. It is a good idea to pair this eating pattern with exercise if you want to reach your ideal weight quickly. It also helps you stay energetic throughout the day.

The Longer Duration Fasting is as follows

The 5:2 Method
In this type of fasting, you can consume regular meals for five days of the week and fast for two days. These two days do not have to be consecutive days of the week. In this method, you can consume some food during the fasting period. This is surprising, isn't it? You can consume up to 500 calories worth of food during your fasting period. It

is always a good idea to consume these calories as one meal on the days you are fasting. This is an effective intermittent fasting method since you can plan your meals in advance. This will help you avoid binging or consuming unhealthy food.

The Alternate Day Fasting

As the name suggests, you will need to fast on alternate days if you want to follow this eating pattern. If you do not want to fast for twenty-four hours, you are allowed to consume 500 calories worth of healthy food. If you feel you can hold it together, then you can follow a strict fast where you consume your regular meals only during your eating period, and consume no food during your fasting period. You may have some hunger pangs and cravings when you follow a strict pattern. When you have such hunger pangs, you can consume beverages like water, tea, green tea, coffee, etc. without sugar.

36 Hour Fasting

In this type of fasting pattern, you can extend or increase your fasting period to thirty-six hours. You will also need to ensure that you consume a few or no calories during your eating period. Your body will, therefore, go through many changes and your cravings may increase. Salt is a medium that the body uses to retain any amount of liquids left in your body, and without salt and sugar based foods your body will need pick me ups that are not processed but are natural. These natural foods will keep you full for longer. Though this form of intermittent fasting is not advisable, patients suffering from diabetes who follow this method of fasting found it to be effective. If you want to teach your body to hold onto insulin for a longer period, you will need to maintain a longer fasting period instead of a shorter fasting period.

>36 Hours Fasting

As the name suggests, you will need to fast for more than 36 hours between your meals. This does not mean that you cannot consume meals during the week. In this pattern, you will need to eat your last meal at 6 p.m., on one day, skip all your meals on the following day and eat breakfast on the third day. This is greater than 36 hours. In this type of fasting, you do not have to restrict your caloric intake since your fasting period is longer than your eating period. If you consume very few calories, you will cause some damage to your body. You may lose your appetite over time if you continue to follow this pattern. This will happen because your body will begin to think that it does not need any food. This will lead to a decrease or lack of appetite.

Chapter Five: How to Choose the Right Method?

It is hard to choose the right pattern since you will need to take many factors into account. You may want to choose a specific pattern because of what someone claims. It is all right to take someone else's experiences into account, but it is a good idea to listen to your body. If you do not listen to your body, it can lead to many illnesses. You should plan the pattern well and ensure that you ease your body into it. Before you dive into choosing the right pattern, ask yourself the following questions.

How Often Do You Eat Healthily?

Yes, this question can be very helpful. You can understand the current state of your body and plan a schedule that will help your body ease into the intermittent fasting schedule. You may wonder why you should worry about eating healthy now when you are following the intermittent fasting pattern to lose weight. You will need to worry about your eating habits because those habits will determine how your body will adjust to change. If you are someone who only consumes junk, you will have withdrawal symptoms. You will find yourself craving for something sweet and salty and will find it hard to control your cravings during the fasting period. Instead of breaking your fast cycle due to some distractions it is always good to control your cravings. This will help you stick to the eating pattern.

How Long Can You Go Without Eating A Meal?
While it may sound ridiculous, hear me out. When was the longest time you went without eating a meal and why? You may not have eaten because you had work or were busy. This means that you are not paying attention to your food habits. When you pay attention to your eating pattern, you can choose the type of intermittent fasting pattern that you want to follow. Since Intermittent Fasting will require a conscious effort, it is important to keep yourself occupied so that you don't give in to your distractions.

How does your schedule look like?
List down the activities you perform on the days you work and on your days-off - at what times you are busy? What days are you off? How many times during the week do you go out with your friends, and so on? This will help you choose the type of fasting method that best suits your needs. Have a cocktail party on the weekend you cannot get away from? Or a Sunday brunch that you love cause you get to spend time with your dear ones? Whatever it

may be, list down everything that is part of your schedule and work around that.

What if I need to go out on a date?

Well, in that case, you will need to plan ahead of time. You can skip your early morning breakfast if you follow the breakfast routine and have that meal for dinner instead. You can then change the pattern and slowly ease your body into the breakfast routine. It can seem a lot in the beginning, but once you start following and prepare your meals in advance, you can address your hunger pangs in a healthy fashion.

Chapter Six: Goal Setting and Tracking Progress

Before diving into your desired intermittent fasting method, it is important to remember that even with all the prep that you did you may notice that this eating pattern does not suit your schedule or your body type. In such cases, take my advice and test the different eating patterns until you identify a pattern that suits you best. In this chapter, we will look at some tips and tricks that can help you set goals and back up plans for when you might have to face a letdown moment.

It is important to remember that it is always the process you follow that makes all the difference. Intermittent Fasting is a way of life, and once you choose this lifestyle, you are in it for the long haul. While it can be very thrilling to see all these results around you, it is important to stop comparing your progress with others. You should always focus on your journey. Here are some ways to keep yourself on track.

Take It Slow
Intermittent Fasting can be tough in the initial stages since you are fasting consciously. This means that a little candy can also be very tempting to you.

That being said, there are cases where people have become obsessed with the diet. To avoid going down that path, you should start small. Only fast when you are sleeping to allow your body to adjust to the pattern. You can gradually increase your fasting period. Ensure that you listen to your body.

Be Consistent

While the word speaks for itself, consistency is the key to the success of any diet that you follow. An extensive form of exercise and intermittent fasting can result in a healthy body and mind. When you are consistent and you track your progress, you can motivate yourself to continue to stick to the pattern. You can track your consistency using various applications. Apps such as meal tracker, habit tracker can help you keep track of your calorie intake.

Eating Quality Food

At any given point having food that is full of nutrients is beneficial for your body when compared to consuming food that lacks nutrition. When you choose to follow this eating pattern, you should keep in mind that you should not consume too many burgers, fries and chips. These will not help you reach your goals. This can also lead you to fall off the wagon as you might say, "What could one burger do?" You must stay strong and control your cravings.

Do Not Overeat

It is important to ensure that you never overeat during your eating period. You should always eat until you are full. If you overeat, you may compensate for the calories that you do not consume during your fasting period. Choose fresh foods such as vegetables, fruits, legumes and good cheese. Such foods not only keep you fuller for longer but also provide your body with the right amount of nutrients it needs.

Chapter Seven: Frequently Asked Questions

In this chapter, I will be answering some of the most asked questions, which can help you make a better choice, and remove any inhibitions before you start this diet.

"Is it recommended to exercise while I'm practicing Intermittent Fasting and, if yes, what kind of exercise do you suggest?"

Yes, absolutely! Pairing exercise with intermittent fasting is the best way to reach your goals. You must remember to take it slow. You can often go overboard because you are in a rush to reach your ideal weight. You forget the pain you put your body through as it is being deprived of its daily dose of food. Your body will soon run out of fuel, which can lead to exhaustion and dizziness. You can choose exercises that can increase your muscle mass by choosing weight-based exercises. Remember that during the first 10 days of your fasting period you may tend to notice a decrease in energy and concentration levels, post which you will tend to pick up the pace and feel easier to exercise. Endurance building exercises such as brisk walking and cycling can increase your stamina and keep you energized throughout the day.

"Will I lose muscle during intermittent fasting?"

It is important to note that all forms of diets will lead to a loss in both muscle and fat. On a regular diet, on an average, you lose 75 % of the fat mass and 25% of the lean mass. In Intermittent Fasting, you lose as little as 10% of the muscle mass. One of the main benefits of intermittent fasting is fat loss, but you must remember that you will also lose muscle in the long run. Pairing your diet with exercise that can build muscle is a good way to avoid loss of muscle. Choosing lean meat and protein-rich food during your fed state is very important to retain your muscle shape and strength.

"Should I continue with fasting if I'm closer to my ideal weight?"

Since it is a lifestyle in itself, it is always a good idea to continue to follow this pattern if you wish to reap all the benefits of intermittent fasting including reduced inflammation, less risk of heart stroke, better immunity and reduced risk of diabetes. If you have lost weight so far, ensure to consume a good amount of calories than before to maintain your weight.

"I'm a snacker, I love to eat snacks throughout the day. Will it be difficult for me to fast?"

Get through the first 10 days. As an individual, you are more susceptible to giving up on the intermittent fasting eating pattern during the first few days. Once you are through the 10-day window, you will find it easier to continue following this eating pattern without any distractions. It is okay to snack on occasion if you are unable to control yourself. Do not be too hard on yourself. You are allowed to give yourself a break from the eating pattern three or four times a month. You should try to drink coffee or tea without sugar when you feel like snacking. You can also choose to drink green tea.

"I just started my intermittent fasting and wanted to know how long it will take for results to show."

Studies show that individuals have lost up to 5 kg in two to three months with a significance level of decrease in insulin levels. Individuals who take up resistance training see significant results of loss in fat with no change in lean/muscle mass. Studies also show that individuals who follow the intermittent fasting eating pattern show a decrease in blood sugar levels at least by three months into the fasting regime.

Conclusion

I sincerely thank you once again for choosing this book. I hope you were able to make an informed decision on the basis of the information in the book.

It always is hard to understand which form of diet is the best one for you. I personally struggled for quite some time to identify mine. Intermittent Fasting is an eating pattern that many people across the world have been following. While intermittent fasting is beneficial, pairing it with low carbs and high protein diets can help to speed up the process.

The power of consistency and hard work in maintaining the effort can lead to gratifying results. Once you get through the first 10 days of the Intermittent Fasting routine and start exercising, it will help you reach your fitness goals in no time and also make you feel exhilarated about the whole process. Maintain a food journal for all your food intakes and have some last minutes recipes up your sleeve. These recipes will save you some time, and maybe effort.

Now that you have all the information you need to start your journey into Intermittent Fasting, I cannot wait to see your results. Be patient, be consistent and don't forget to have fun.

Finally, if you enjoyed this book, then I'd like to ask you for a favor, would you be kind enough to **leave**

a review for this book on Amazon? It would be very much appreciated!

Thank you and good luck!

Sources

https://www.healthline.com/nutrition/intermittent-fasting-guide

https://www.dietdoctor.com/intermittent-fasting

https://www.precisionnutrition.com/intermittent-fasting-women

https://www.bodyandsoul.com.au/nutrition/nutrition-tips/the-6-people-who-shouldnt-try-intermittent-fasting-according-to-a-dietitian/news-story/ca97f74fc904811f4b78281824dea72c

www.ingramcontent.com/pod-product-compliance
Lightning Source LLC
Chambersburg PA
CBHW051406280526
45784CB00007B/3120